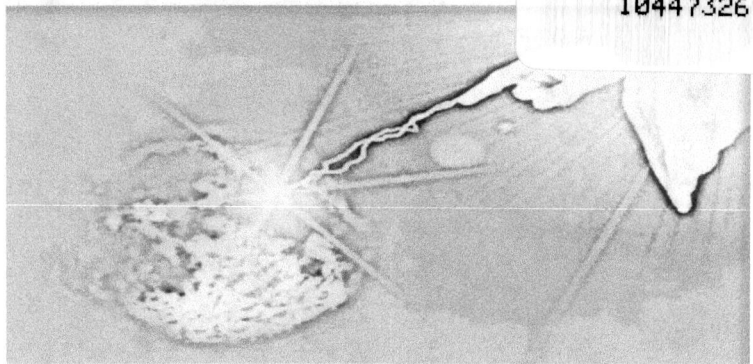

Iniquity and Infidelity, the Destroyers of Man

By Rev. Melissa Smith

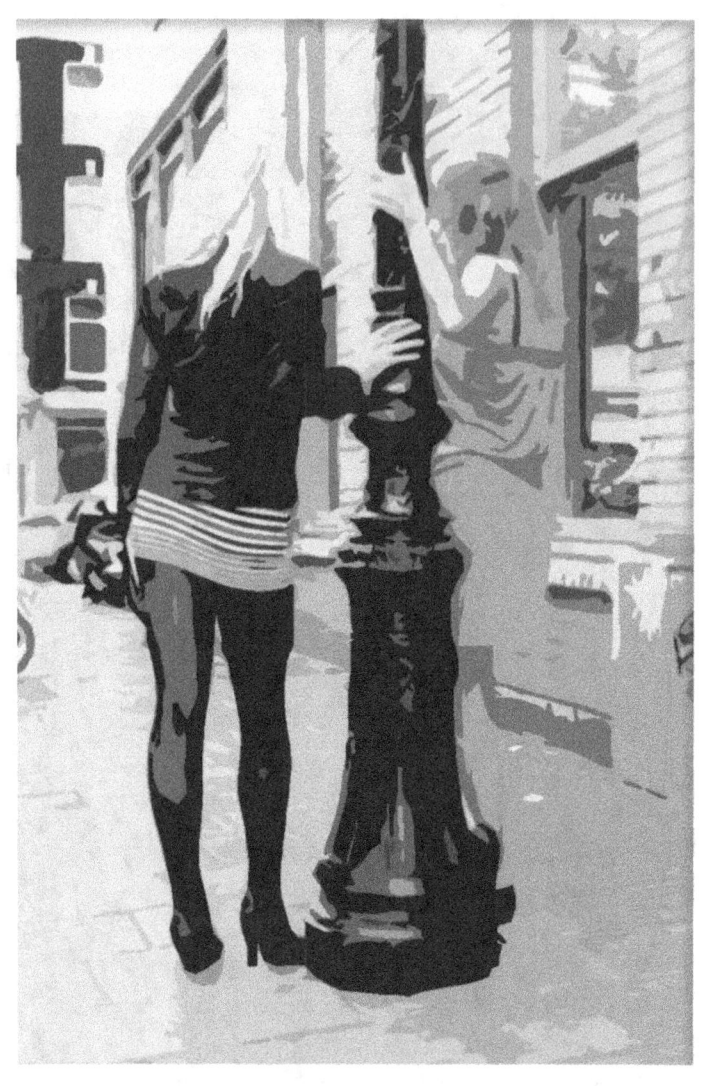

Copyright Prohibited

2012

'Keep a sure watch over a shameless daughter, lest at any time she make thee become a laughing stock to thy enemies, and a by word in the city, and a reproach among the people, and she make thee ashamed before all the multitude.

Behold not everybody's beauty and tarry not among women. For from garments cometh a moth, and from a woman the iniquity of a man.'

Yeshua Ben Sira, Ch. 42
Verses 11-13

INTRODUCTION

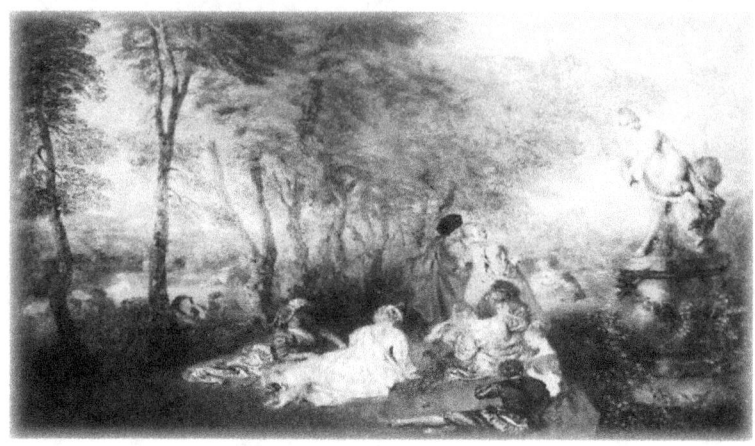

Throughout the ages, on every continent, among every people of the Earth infidelity and sex have been at the center of most major travesties that have been the corruptor of people and the destroyer of nations.

Infidelity and iniquity partnered together is much like having been diagnosed with a terminal illness for you, your family and love ones. Like the diagnosis given, it is oftentimes received in fear of one's physical mortality and death.

Per Webster's 1828 Dictionary, infidelity is defined as the following:

INFIDEL'ITY, noun

1. In general, want of faith or belief; a withholding of credit.

2. Disbelief of the inspiration of the Scriptures, or the divine original of christianity; unbelief.

3. Unfaithfulness, particularly in married persons; a violation of the marriage covenant by adultery or lewdness.

4. Breach of trust; treachery; deceit; as the infidelity of a friend or a servant. In this sense, unfaithfulness is most used.

The etymology of the word, "infidelity" requires a further examination of "infidel" and it's meaning.

From the same dictionary, Webster's 1828 Dictionary, infidel is defined as the following:

IN'FIDEL, a.

Unbelieving; disbelieving the inspiration of the Scriptures, or the divine institution of christianity.

The infidel writer is a great enemy to society.

IN'FIDEL, n.

One who disbelieves the inspiration of the Scriptures, and the divine origin of christianity.

INIQ'UITY, n

1. Injustice; unrighteousness; a deviation from rectitude; as the iniquity of war; the

iniquity of the slave trade.

2. Want of rectitude in principle; as a malicious prosecution originating in the iniquity of the author.

3. A particular deviation from rectitude; a sin or crime; wickedness; any act of injustice.

4. Original want of holiness or depravity.

Finally, the ending, "ity" requires defining:

'ITY, suffix meaning the character, state or condition of being

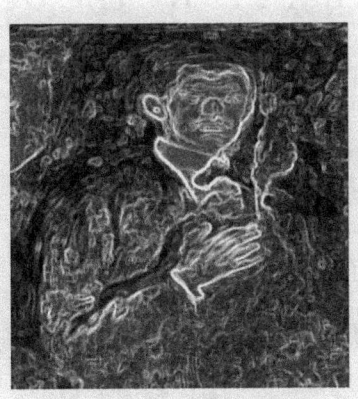

In this case, the illness is two-fold, "iniquity and infidelity." For many, it is only when the medical condition is known that all avenues of treatment are sought.

Success in treatment resulting in a complete cure and remission of the disease does not come to all.

9

The goal of this work is to assist you in recognizing the affects on your personal, physical, financial and spiritual life by the destroyer infidelity and its partner infidelity that they be easily avoided.

May your wisdom be increased for the betterment of your life.

Rev. Melissa Smith

You have been presented with the premise that iniquity partnered with infidelity is an enemy to man in essence, to you.

In order to know just how this is so, let us take a look at the definition of the word, "enemy."

Again referencing the 1828 Webster's Dictionary, the meaning of enemy:

EN'EMY, n.

> 1. A foe, an adversary. A private enemy is one who hates another and wishes him injury, or attempts to do him

injury to gratify his own malice or ill will. A public enemy or foe, is one who belongs to a nation or party, at war with another.

2. One who hates or dislikes; as an enemy to truth or falsehood.

3. In theology, and by way of eminence, the enemy is the Devil; the archfiend.

4. In military affairs, the opposing army or naval force in war, is called the enemy.

Hence, the intent of an enemy is to "do YOU HARM." To bring about an injury to and upon you. The injuries bought about by iniquity and infidelity are detrimental to every aspect of your life and if you or someone you know have partaken of these bitter activities then it is time to illustrate to you how you became a victim, was injured and the solution to your healing.

In your life, the following are manipulated to weaken you:

1. Senses
2. Visualization
3. Sexuality

How you ask?

Throughout the ages, the true knowledge of the being and origin of man was removed or rather hidden and was replaced with partial truths mixed with fictional information.

Thus commencing the implementation of the negative "Social Engineering" of man.

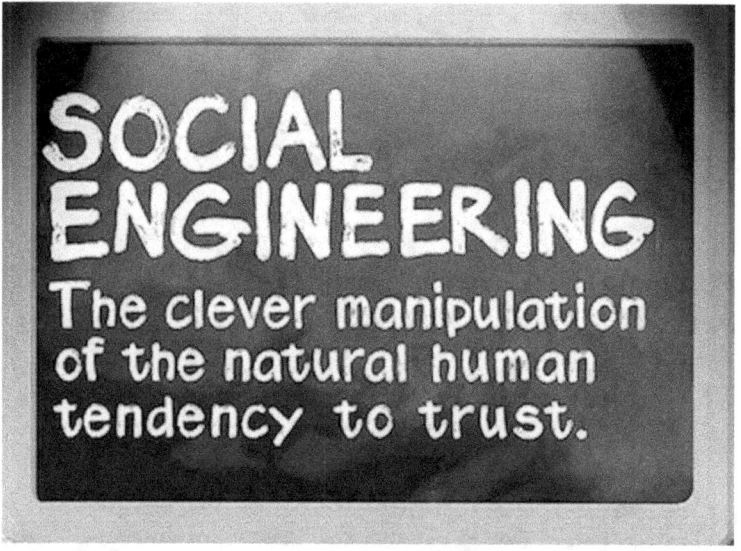

Whereby, lies were taught as truths and truths were observed as lies and untrue. Hence, social engineering can be viewed as a weapon and was used to harm you.

Another dangerous weapon that was used to harm you was the invention and implementation of "genetically modified foods."

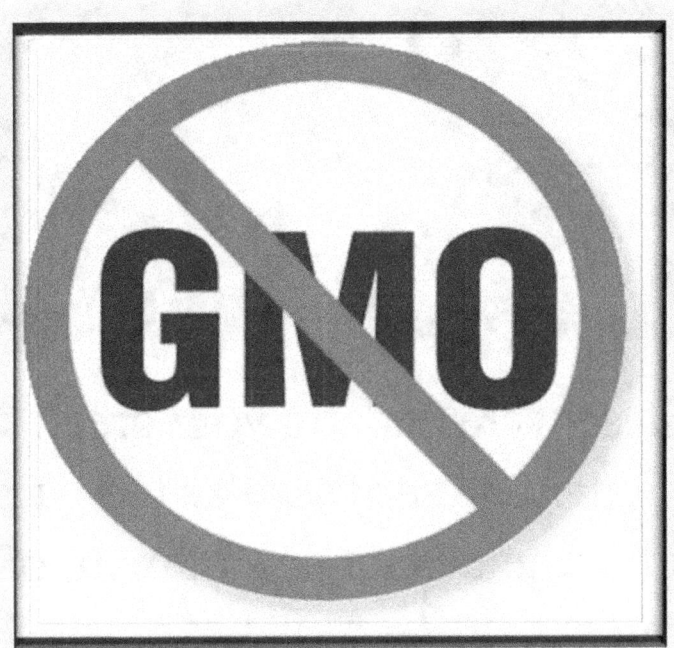

With the genetic modification of foods for man, it resulted in the greatest success for your unseen and unknown enemy, the "altering of your DNA."

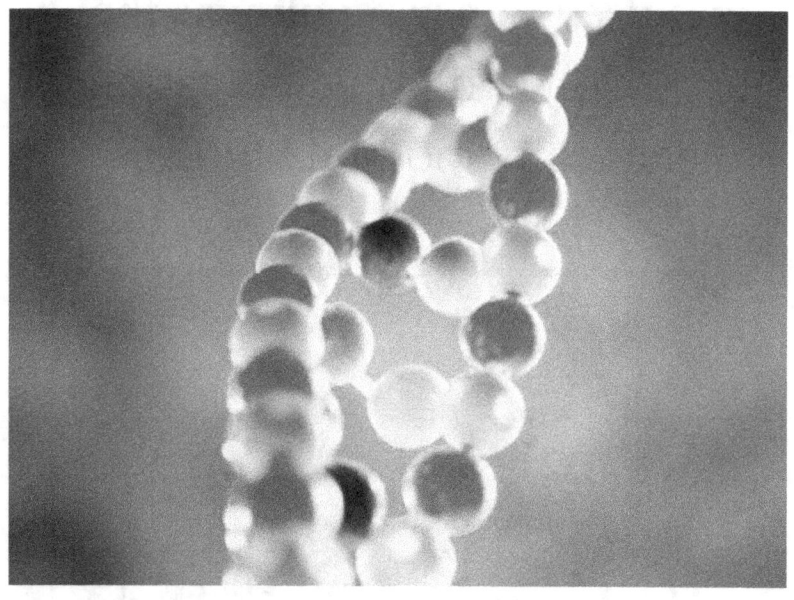

These were and are your greatest enemies and are used as tools to aid in the destruction of man, of you.

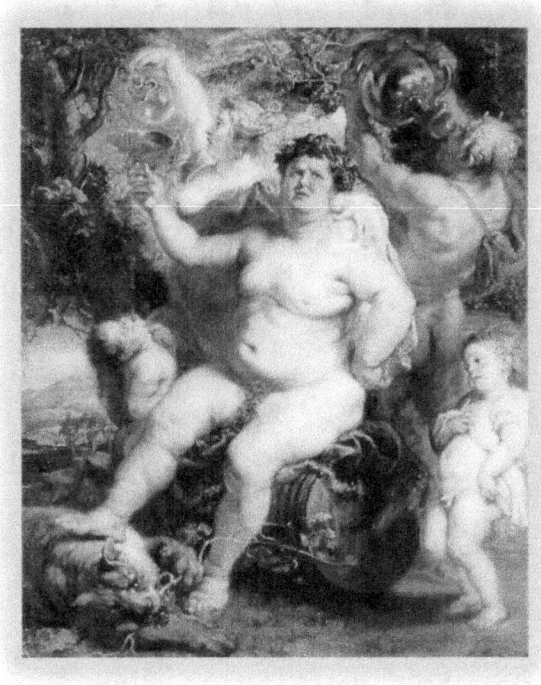

From youth, the Roman demigod, Bacchus has been a major corruptor of man with his elixirs of intoxication.

Over 2,000 years ago, in two ancient scrolls collected and hidden from man, the "Gospel of

Peace" and the "Gospel of the Holy Twelve" were the instructions and teachings of Christ that included the following commandment:

To abstain from any food or drink that "disrupted" your health or senses.

Wines, liquors, spirits easily available throughout the Earth all have been created, mixed together and administered to men and women alike with the same end results of promiscuity, fornication, adultery, infidel behavior, violence and even murder.

The weapon that has been the most profitable in the destroying of man is the visualizations of intimacies and sex.

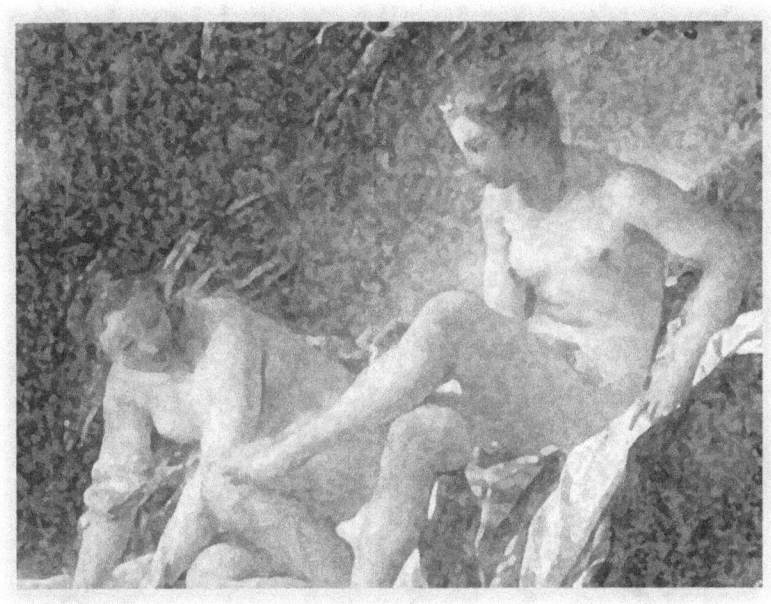

In ancient days, a simple act of bathing in a lake or stream was the norm and nudity was not seen as being bad and perverse. However, over time the people of the world were engineered into thinking otherwise. Thus, began the sexualization of man.

At every turn, man was bombarded with sexual imagery.

In art, books, media sex became an overnight success.

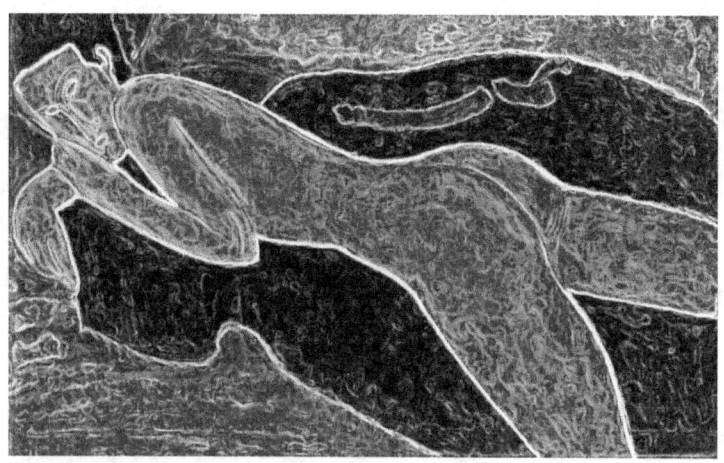

Leading to the nuclear weapon "Pornography" and the full on assault against man.

Since the development of pornography, more diversive weapons have been included in the artillery of iniquity and infidelity. Some of these being:

1. Social Media
2. Online Dating
3. Technology

Intimate diversions mixed with technological tools i.e. gps, iphone, ipad makes for an easy coming together of iniquity and infidelity.

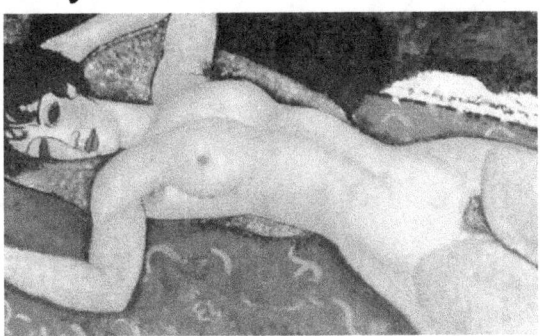

In order for you to win the assault of iniquity, you must become aware and familiar with the teachings of ancient's past that you might have a better today and a brighter future.

Why? It is necessary for your success.

From the very beginning of man's existence upon Earth, he was told throughout the ages to live righteously and to seek wisdom that his days might be long.

Therefore the key to your succeeding is linked to wisdom.

However, King Solomon in his "Book of Wisdom" firmly states, "that where iniquity abides, wisdom cannot dwell."

Thus, you were until this moment was unaware of the link between iniquity and wisdom.

When one leads a life of iniquity, wisdom is not present therefore, infidelity creeps in and is allowed to take root causing one to live unrighteously and to your detriment.

Wisdom was created for man. Iniquity and infidelity was created against man.

BOOK OF WISDOM

Love justice, you that are the judges of the earth. Think of the Lord in goodness, and seek him in simplicity of heart.

For he is found by them that tempt him not: and he sheweth himself to them that have faith in him.

For perverse thoughts separate from God and his power, when it is tried, reproveth the unwise.

For wisdom will not enter into a malicious soul, nor dwell in a body subject to sins.

For the Holy Spirit of discipline will flee from the deceitful, and will withdraw himself from thoughts that are without understanding, and he shall not abide when iniquity cometh in.

For the spirit of wisdom is benevolent, and will not acquit the evil speaker from his lips.

For God is witness of his reins, and he is a true searcher of his heart, and a hearer of his tongue.

For the spirit of the Lord hath filled the whole world: and that, which containeth all things, hath knowledge of the voice.

Therefore he that speaketh unjust things cannot be hid, neither shall the chastising judgment pass him by.

For inquisition shall be made into the thoughts of the ungodly and the hearing of his words shall come to God, to the chastising of his iniquities.

For the ear of jealousy heareth all things, and the tumult of murmuring shall not be hid.

Keep yourselves therefore from murmuring, which profiteth nothing, and refrain your tongue from detraction, for an obscure speech shall not go for nought and the mouth that be lieth, killeth the soul.

Seek not death in the error of your life, neither procure ye destruction by the works of your hands.

For God made not death, neither hath he pleasure in the destruction of the living.

For he created all things that they might be and he made the nations of the earth for health and there is no poison of destruction in them, nor kingdom of hell upon the earth.

For justice is perpetual and immortal.

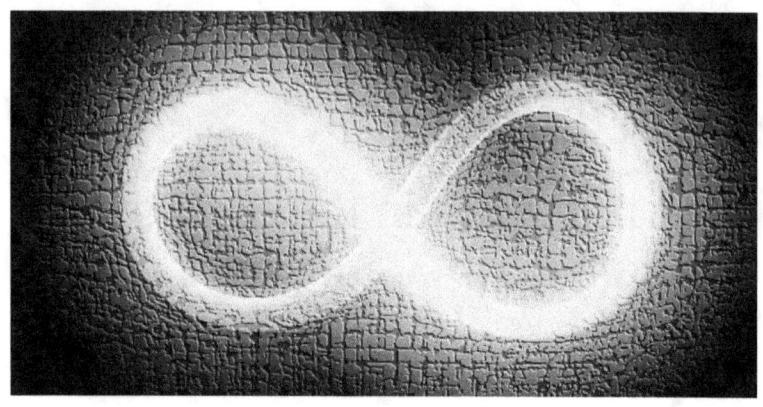

But the wicked with works and words have called it to them: and esteeming it a friend have fallen away, and have made a covenant with it because they are worthy to be of the part thereof.

Chapter 2

For they have said, reasoning with themselves, but not right. The time of our life is short and tedious, and in the end of a man there is no remedy, and no man hath been known to have returned from hell.

For we are born of nothing, and after this we shall be as if we had not been for the breath in our nostrils is smoke: and speech a spark to move our heart.

Which being put out, our body shall be ashes, and our spirit shall be poured abroad as soft air, and our life shall pass away as the trace of a cloud, and shall be dispersed as a mist, which is driven away by the beams of the sun, and overpowered with the heat thereof and our name in time shall be forgotten, and no man shall have any remembrance of our works.

For our time is as the passing of a shadow, and there is no going back of our end: for it is fast sealed, and no man returneth.

Come therefore, and let us enjoy the good things that are present, and let us speedily use the creatures as in youth.

Let us fill ourselves with costly wine, and ointments and let not the flower of the time pass by us. Let us crown ourselves with roses, before they be withered, let no meadow escape our riot.

Let none of us go without his part in luxury, let us everywhere leave tokens of joy for this is our portion, and this our lot.

Let us oppress the poor just man, and not spare the widow, nor honour the ancient grey hairs of the aged.

But let our strength be the law of justice: for that which is feeble, is found to be nothing worth.

Let us therefore lie in wait for the just, because he is not for our turn, and he is contrary to our doings, and upbraideth us with transgressions of the law, and divulgeth against us the sins of our way of life.

He boasteth that he hath the knowledge of God, and calleth himself the son of God.

He is become a censurer of our thoughts. He is grievous unto us, even to behold for his life is not like other men's, and his ways are very different.

We are esteemed by him as triflers, and he abstaineth from our ways as from filthiness, and he preferreth the latter end of the just, and glorieth that he hath God for his father.

Let us see then if his words be true, and let us prove what shall happen to him, and we shall know what his end shall be.

For if he be the true son of God, he will defend him, and will deliver him from the hands of his enemies.

Let us examine him by outrages and tortures, that we may know his meekness and try his patience.

Let us condemn him to a most shameful death for there shall be respect had unto him by his words.

These things they thought, and were deceived for their own malice blinded them.

And they knew not the secrets of God, nor hoped for the wages of justice, nor esteemed the honour of holy souls.

For God created man incorruptible, and to the image of his own likeness he made him.

But by the envy of the devil, death came into the world they follow him that are of his side.

Chapter 3

But the souls of the just are in the hand of God, and the torment of death shall not touch them. In the sight of the unwise they seemed to die: and their departure was taken for misery.

And their going away from us, for utter destruction but they are in peace.

And though in the sight of men they suffered torments, their hope is full of immortality. Afflicted in few things, in many they shall be well rewarded because God hath tried them, and found them worthy of himself.

As gold in the furnace he hath proved them, and as a victim of a holocaust he hath received them, and in time there shall be respect had to them.

The just shall shine, and shall run to and fro like sparks among the reeds. They shall judge nations, and rule over people, and their Lord shall reign forever. They that trust in him, shall understand the truth and they that are faithful in love shall rest in him.

For grace and peace is to his elect. But the wicked shall be punished according to their own devices: who have neglected the just, and have revolted from the Lord.

For he that rejecteth wisdom, and discipline, is unhappy and their hope is vain, and their labours without fruit, and their works unprofitable.

Their wives are foolish, and their children wicked. Their offspring is cursed: for happy is the barren and the undefiled, that hath not known bed in sin, she shall have fruit in the visitation of holy souls.

And the eunuch, that hath not wrought iniquity with his hands, nor thought wicked things against God.

For the precious gift of faith shall be given to him, and a most acceptable lot in the temple of God.

For the fruit of good labours is glorious, and the root of wisdom never faileth.

But the children of adulterers shall not come to perfection, and the seed of the unlawful bed shall be rooted out.

And if they live long, they shall be nothing regarded, and their last old age shall be without honour.

And if they die quickly, they shall have no hope, nor speech of comfort in the day of trial.

For dreadful are the ends of a wicked race.

Chapter 4

O how beautiful is the chaste generation with glory for the memory thereof is immortal because it is known both with God and with men.

When it is present, they imitate it and they desire it when it hath withdrawn itself, and it triumpheth crowned forever, winning the reward of undefiled conflicts.

But the multiplied brood of the wicked shall not thrive, and shall not take deep root, nor any fast foundation.

And if they flourish in branches for a time, yet standing not fast, they shall be shaken with the wind, and through the force of winds they shall be rooted out.

For the branches not being perfect, shall be broken and their fruits shall be unprofitable, sour to eat and fit for nothing.

For the children that are born of unlawful beds, are witnesses of wickedness against their parents in their trial.

But the just man, if he be prevented with death, shall be in rest. For venerable old age is not that of long time, nor counted by the number of years: but the understanding of a man is grey hairs.

And a spotless life is old age. He pleased God and was beloved, and living among sinners he was translated.

He was taken away lest wickedness should alter his understanding, or deceit beguile his soul.

For the bewitching of vanity obscureth good things, and the

wandering of concupiscence over turneth the innocent mind.

Being made perfect in a short space, he fulfilled a long time for his soul pleased God therefore he hastened to bring him out of the midst of iniquities.

But the people see this, and understand not, nor lay up such things in their hearts that the grace of God, and his mercy is with his saints and that he hath respect to his chosen.

But the just that is dead, condemneth the wicked that are living, and youth soon ended, the long life of the unjust.

For they shall see the end of the wise man, and shall not understand what God hath designed for him, and why the Lord hath set him in safety.

They shall see him, and shall despise him: but the Lord shall laugh them to scorn.

And they shall fall after this without honour and be a reproach among the dead for ever: for he shall burst them puffed up and speechless, and shall shake them from the foundations, and they shall be utterly laid waste they shall be in sorrow, and their memory shall perish.

They shall come with fear at the thought of their sins, and their iniquities shall stand against them to convict them.

Chapter 5

Then shall the just stand with great constancy against those that have afflicted them, and taken away their labours. These seeing it, shall be troubled with terrible fear, and shall be amazed at the suddenness of their unexpected salvation.

Saying within themselves, repenting, and groaning for anguish of spirit. These are they, whom we had some time in derision, and for a parable of reproach. We fools esteemed their life madness, and their end without honour.

Behold how they are numbered among the children of God, and their lot is among the saints.

Therefore we have erred from the way of truth, and the light of justice hath not shined unto us, and the sun of understanding hath not risen upon us.

We wearied ourselves in the way of iniquity and destruction, and have walked through hard ways, but the way of the Lord we have not known.

What hath pride profited us? Or what advantage hath the boasting of riches brought us?

All those things are passed away like a shadow, and like a post that runneth on and as a ship that passeth through the waves whereof when it is gone by, the trace cannot be found, nor the path of its keel in the waters.

Or as when a bird flieth through the air, of the passage of which no mark can be found, but only the sound of the wings beating the light air, and parting it by the force of her flight; she moved her wings, and hath flown through, and there is no mark found afterwards of her way.

Or as when an arrow is shot at a mark, the divided air presently cometh together again, so that the passage thereof is not known.

So we also being born, forthwith ceased to be and have been able to shew no mark of virtue but are consumed in our wickedness.

Such things as these the sinners said in hell.

For the hope of the wicked is as dust, which is blown away with the wind, and as a thin froth which is dispersed by the storm and a smoke that is scattered abroad by the wind and as the remembrance of a guest of one day that passeth by.

But the just shall live for evermore and their reward is with the Lord, and the care of them with the most High.

Therefore shall they receive a kingdom of glory, and a crown of beauty at the hand of the Lord: for with his right hand he will cover them, and with his holy arm he will defend them.

And his zeal will take armour, and he will arm the creature for the revenge of his enemies. He will put on justice as a breastplate, and will take true judgment instead of a helmet. He will take equity for an invincible shield:

And he will sharpen his severe wrath for a spear, and the whole world shall fight with him against the unwise.

Then shafts of lightning shall go directly from the clouds, as from a bow well bent, they shall be shot out, and shall fly to the mark.

And thick hail shall be cast upon them from the stone casting wrath: the water of the sea shall rage against them, and the rivers shall run together in a terrible manner.

A mighty wind shall stand up against them, and as a whirlwind shall divide them and their iniquity shall bring all the earth to a desert, and wickedness shall overthrow the thrones of the mighty.

Chapter 6

Wisdom is better than strength, and a wise man is better than a strong man.

Hear therefore, ye kings, and understand: learn, ye that are judges of the ends of the earth.

Give ear, you that rule the people, and that please yourselves in multitudes of nations.

For power is given you by the Lord, and strength by the most High, who will examine your works, and search out your thoughts.

Because being ministers of his kingdom, you have not judged rightly, nor kept the law of justice, nor walked according to the will of God.

Horribly and speedily will he appear to you for a most severe judgment shall be for them that bear rule.

For to him that is little, mercy is granted but the mighty shall be mightily tormented.

For God will not except any man's person, neither will he stand in awe of any man's greatness for he made the little and the great, and he hath equally care of all. But a greater punishment is ready for the more mighty.

To you, therefore, O kings, are these my words, that you may learn wisdom, and not fall from it.

For they that have kept just things justly, shall be justified: and they that have learned these things, shall find what to answer.

Covet ye therefore my words, and love them, and you shall have instruction.

Wisdom is glorious, and never fadeth away, and is easily seen by them that love her, and is found by them that seek her.

She preventeth them that covet her, so that she first sheweth herself unto them.

He that awaketh early to seek her, shall not labour for he shall find her sitting at his door.

To think therefore upon her, is perfect understanding and he that watcheth for her, shall quickly be secure.

For she goeth about seeking such as are worthy of her, and she sheweth herself to them cheerfully in the ways, and meeteth them with all providence.

For the beginning of her is the most true desire of discipline.

And the care of discipline is love: and love is the keeping of her laws: and the keeping of her laws is the firm foundation of incorruption

And incorruption bringeth near to God.

Therefore the desire of wisdom bringeth to the everlasting kingdom.

If then your delight be in thrones, and sceptres, o ye kings of the people, love wisdom, that you may reign forever.

Love the light of wisdom, all ye that bear rule over peoples.

Now what wisdom is, and what was her origin, I will declare and I will not hide from you the mysteries of God, but will seek her out from the beginning of her birth, and bring the knowledge of her to light, and will not pass over the truth.

Neither will I go with consuming envy for such a man shall not be partaker of wisdom.

Now the multitude of the wise is the welfare of the whole world: and a wise king is the upholding of the people.

Receive therefore instruction by my words, and it shall be profitable to you.

Chapter 7

I myself also am a mortal man, like all others, and of the race of him, that was first made of the earth, and in the womb of my mother I was fashioned to be flesh.

In the time of ten months I was compacted in blood, of the seed of man, and the pleasure of sleep concurring. And being born I drew in the common air, and fell upon the earth, that is made alike, and the first voice which I uttered was crying, as all others do. I was nursed in swaddling clothes, and with great cares.

For none of the kings had any other beginning of birth.

For all men have one entrance into life, and the like going out.

Wherefore I wished, and understanding was given me: and I called upon God, and the spirit of wisdom came upon me and I preferred her before kingdoms and thrones, and esteemed riches nothing in comparison of her.

Neither did I compare unto her any precious stone: for all gold in comparison of her, is as a little sand, and silver in respect to her shall be counted as clay.

I loved her above health and beauty, and chose to have her instead of light for her light cannot be put out.

Now all good things came to me together with her, and innumerable riches through her hands and I rejoiced in all these for this wisdom went before me and I knew not that she was the mother of them all.

Which I have learned without guile, and communicate without envy, and her riches I hide not.

For she is an infinite treasure to men! which they that use, become the friends of God, being commended for the gift of discipline.

And God hath given to me to speak as I would, and to conceive thoughts worthy of those things that are given me because he is the guide of wisdom and the director of the wise.

For in his hand are both we, and our words, and all wisdom, and the knowledge and skill of works.

For he hath given me the true knowledge of the things that are: to know the disposition of the whole world, and the virtues of the elements.

The beginning and ending, and midst of the times, the alterations of their courses and the changes of seasons, the revolutions of the year, and the dispositions of the stars, the natures of living creatures, and rage of wild beasts, the force of winds, and reasonings of men, the diversities of plants, and the virtues of roots,

And all such things as are hid and not foreseen, I have learned for wisdom, which is the worker of all things, taught me.

For in her is the spirit of understanding holy, one, manifold, subtile, eloquent, active, undefiled, sure, sweet, loving that which is good, quick, which nothing hindereth, beneficent, gentle, kind, steadfast, assured, secure, having all power, overseeing all things, and containing all spirits, intelligible, pure, subtile.

For wisdom is more active than all active things and reacheth everywhere by reason of her purity.

For she is a vapour of the power of God and a certain pure emanation of the glory of the almighty God and therefore no defiled thing cometh into her.

For she is the brightness of eternal light and the unspotted mirror of God's majesty and the image of his goodness.

And being but one, she can do all things and remaining in herself the same, she reneweth all things, and through nations conveyeth herself into holy souls, she maketh the friends of God and prophets.

For God loveth none but him that dwelleth with wisdom.

For she is more beautiful than the sun, and above all the order of the stars being compared with the light, she is found before it.

For after this cometh night, but no evil can overcome wisdom.

Chapter 8

She reacheth therefore from end to end mightily and ordereth all things sweetly. Her have I loved, and have sought her out from my youth and have desired to take her for my spouse and I became a lover of her beauty.

She glorifieth her nobility by being conversant with God yea and the Lord of all things hath loved her.

For it is she that teacheth the knowledge of God and is the chooser of his works.

And if riches be desired in life, what is richer than wisdom, which maketh all things?

And if sense do work, who is a more artful worker than she of those things that are?

And if a man love justice her labours have great virtues, for she teacheth temperance, prudence, justice and fortitude, which are such things as men can have nothing more profitable in life.

And if a man desire much knowledge she knoweth things past and judgeth of things to come, she knoweth the subtilties of speeches, and the solutions of arguments, she knoweth signs and wonders before they be done, and the events of times and ages.

I purposed therefore to take her to me to live with me, knowing that she will communicate to me of her good things, and will be a comfort in my cares and grief.

For her sake I shall have glory among the multitude, and honour with the ancients, though I be young:

And I shall be found of a quick conceit in judgment, and shall be admired in the sight of the mighty, and the faces of princes shall wonder at me.

They shall wait for me when I hold my peace, and they shall look upon me when I speak, and if I talk much they shall lay their hands on their mouths.

Moreover by the means of her I shall have immortality and shall leave behind me an everlasting memory to them that come after me.

I shall set the people in order and nations shall be subject to me. Terrible kings hearing shall be afraid of me: among the multitude I shall be found good, and valiant in war.

When I go into my house, I shall repose myself with her: for her conversation hath no bitterness, nor her company any tediousness, but joy and gladness.

Thinking these things with myself, and pondering them in my heart, that to be allied to wisdom is immortality and that there is great delight in her friendship, and inexhaustible riches in the works of her hands, and in the exercise of conference with her, wisdom, and glory in the communication of her words.

I went about seeking, that I might take her to myself. And I was a witty child and had received a good soul.

And whereas I was more good, I came to a body undefiled.

And as I knew that I could not otherwise be continent, except God gave it, and this also was a point of wisdom, to know whose gift it was: I went to the Lord, and besought him, and said with my whole heart:

Chapter 9

God of my fathers, and Lord of mercy, who hast made all things with thy word and by thy wisdom hast appointed man, that he should have dominion over the creature that was made by thee.

That he should order the world according to equity and justice and execute justice with an upright heart. Give me wisdom, that sitteth by thy throne and cast me not off from among thy children

For I am thy servant and the son of thy handmaid, a weak man, and of short time, and falling short of the understanding of judgment and laws.

For if one be perfect among the children of men, yet if thy wisdom be not with him, he shall be nothing regarded.

Thou hast chosen me to be king of thy people and a judge of thy sons and daughters. And hast commanded me to build a temple on thy holy mount, and an altar in the city of thy dwelling place, a resemblance of thy holy tabernacle, which thou hast prepared from the beginning.

And thy wisdom with thee, which knoweth thy works, which then also was present when thou madest the world and knew what was agreeable to thy eyes and what was right in thy commandments.

Send her out of thy holy heaven, and from the throne of thy majesty, that she may be with me, and may labour with me, that I may know what is acceptable with thee.

For she knoweth and understandeth all things and shall lead me soberly in my works, and shall preserve me by her power.

So shall my works be acceptable and I shall govern thy people justly, and shall be worthy of the throne of my father.

For who among men is he that can know the counsel of God? Or who can think what the will of God is?

For the thoughts of mortal men are fearful and our counsels uncertain.

For the corruptible body is a load upon the soul, and the earthly habitation presseth down the mind that museth upon many things.

And hardly do we guess aright at things that are upon earth and with labour do we find the things that are before us.

But the things that are in heaven, who shall search out? And who shall know thy thought, except thou give wisdom, and send thy Holy Spirit from above.

And so the ways of them that are upon earth may be corrected, and men may learn the things that please thee?

For by wisdom they were healed, whosoever have pleased thee, O Lord, from the beginning.

Chapter 10

She preserved him, that was first formed by God the father of the world, when he was created alone.

And she brought him out of his sin, and gave him power to govern all things.

But when the unjust went away from her in his anger, he perished by the fury wherewith he murdered his brother.

For whose cause, when water destroyed the earth, wisdom

healed it again, directing the course of the just by contemptible wood.

Moreover when the nations had conspired together to consent to wickedness, she knew the just and preserved him without blame to God, and kept him strong against the compassion for his son.

She delivered the just man who fled from the wicked that were perishing, when the fire came down upon Pentapolis (Sodom, Gomorrha, Segor also known as Zoar, Adama and Seboim.

Whose land for a testimony of their wickedness is desolate, and smoketh to this day, and the trees bear fruits that ripen not, and a standing pillar of salt is a monument of an incredulous soul.

For regarding not wisdom, they did not only slip in this, that they were ignorant of good things, but they left also unto men a memorial of their folly, so that in the things in which they sinned, they could not so much as lie hid.

But wisdom hath delivered from sorrow them that attend upon her. She conducted the just, when he fled from his brother's wrath, through the right ways and shewed him the kingdom of God, and gave him the knowledge of the holy things, made him honourable in his labours and accomplished his labours.

In the deceit of them that overreached him, she stood by him, and made him honourable.

] She kept him safe from his enemies, and she defended him from seducers, and gave him a strong conflict, that he might overcome, and know that wisdom is mightier than all.

She forsook not the just when he was sold, but delivered him from sinners, she went down with him into the pit. And in bands she left him not, till she brought him the sceptre of the kingdom, and power against those that oppressed him and shewed them to be liars that had accused him, and gave him everlasting glory.

She delivered the just people, and blameless seed from the nations that oppressed them.

She entered into the soul of the servant of God and stood against dreadful kings in wonders and signs.

And she rendered to the just the wages of their labours, and conducted them in a wonderful way: and she was to them for a covert by day, and for the light of stars by night.

And she brought them through the Red Sea, and carried them over through a great water. But their enemies she drowned in the sea, and from the depth of hell she brought them out.

Therefore the just took the spoils of the wicked. And they sung to thy holy name, O Lord, and they praised with one accord thy victorious hand.

For wisdom opened the mouth of the dumb, and made the tongues of infants eloquent.

Chapter 11

She prospered their works in the hands of the holy prophet. They went through wildernesses that were not inhabited and in desert places they pitched their tents.

They stood against their enemies, and revenged themselves of their adversaries.

They were thirsty and they called upon thee, and water was given them out of the high rock, and a refreshment of their thirst out of the hard stone.

For by what things their enemies were punished, when their drink failed them, while the children of Israel abounded therewith and rejoiced.

By the same things they in their need were benefited. For instead of a fountain of an ever running river, thou gavest human blood to the unjust.

And whilst they were diminished for a manifest reproof of their murdering the infants, thou gavest to thine abundant water unlooked for shewing by the thirst that was then, how thou didst exalt thine and didst kill their adversaries. For when they were tried and chastised with mercy, they knew how the wicked were judged with wrath and tormented.

For thou didst admonish and try them as a father but the others, as a severe king, thou didst examine and condemn. For whether absent or present, they were tormented alike.

For a double affliction came upon them, and a groaning for the remembrance of things past.

For when they heard that by their punishments the others were benefited, they remembered the Lord, wondering at the end of what was come to pass. For whom they scorned before, when he was thrown out at the time of his being wickedly exposed to perish, him they admired in the end, when they saw the event, their thirsting being unlike to that of the just.

But for the foolish devices of their iniquity, because some being deceived worshipped dumb serpents and worthless beasts, thou didst send upon them a multitude of dumb beasts for vengeance.

That they might know that by what things a man sinneth, by the same also he is tormented.

For thy almighty hand, which made the world of matter without form, was not unable to send upon them a multitude of bears, or fierce lions.

Or unknown beasts of a new kind, full of rage either breathing out a fiery vapour, or sending forth a stinking smoke, or shooting horrible sparks out of their eyes.

Whereof not only the hurt might be able to destroy them, but also the very sight might kill them through fear.

Yea and without these, they might have been slain with one

blast, persecuted by their own deeds, and scattered by the breath of thy power but, thou hast ordered all things in measure, and number, and weight.

For great power always belonged to thee alone: and who shall resist the strength of thy arm?

For the whole world before thee is as the least grain of the balance, and as a drop of the morning dew, that falleth down upon the earth.

But thou hast mercy upon all, because thou canst do all things, and over lookest the sins of men for the sake of repentance.

For thou lovest all things that are, and hatest none of the things which thou hast made: for thou didst not appoint, or make any thing hating it.

And how could any thing endure, if thou wouldst not? Or be preserved, if not called by thee.

But thou sparest all because they are thine, O Lord, who lovest souls.

Chapter 12

O how good and sweet is thy spirit, O Lord, in all things!

And therefore thou chastisest them that err, by little and little and admonishest them, and speakest to them, concerning the things wherein they offend: that leaving their wickedness, they may believe in thee, O Lord.

For those ancient inhabitants of thy holy land, whom thou didst abhor.

Because they did works hateful to thee by their sorceries, and wicked sacrifices and those merciless murderers of their own children, and eaters of men's bowels, and devourers of blood from the midst of thy consecration, from the midst of thy consecration.

And those parents sacrificing with their own hands helpless souls, it was thy will to destroy by the hands of our parents.

That the land which of all is most dear to thee might receive a worthy colony of the children of God.

Yet even those thou sparedst as men, and didst send wasps, forerunners of thy host, to destroy them by little and little.

Not that thou wast unable to bring the wicked under the just by war, or by cruel beasts, or with one rough word to destroy them at once.

But executing thy judgments by degrees thou gavest them place of repentance, not being ignorant that they were a wicked generation, and their malice natural, and that their thought could never be changed.

For it was a cursed seed from the beginning neither didst thou for fear of any one give pardon to their sins.

For who shall say to thee: What hast thou done? Or who shall withstand thy judgment? Or who shall come before thee to be a revenger of wicked men? Or who shall accuse thee if, the nations perish, which thou hast made?

For there is no other God but thou, who hast care of all, that thou shouldst shew that thou dost not give judgment unjustly.

Neither shall king, nor tyrant in thy sight inquire about them whom thou hast destroyed.

For so much then as thou art just, thou orderest all things justly, thinking it not agreeable to thy power, to condemn him who deserveth not to be punished.

For thy power is the beginning of justice and because thou art Lord of all, thou makest thyself gracious to all.

For thou shewest thy power, when men will not believe thee to be absolute in power, and thou convincest the boldness of them that know thee not.

But thou being master of power, judgest with tranquillity and with great favour disposest of us for thy power is at hand when thou wilt.

But thou hast taught thy people by such works, that they must be just and humane, and hast made thy children to be of a good hope: because in judging thou givest place for repentance for sins.

For if thou didst punish the enemies of thy servants, and that deserved to die, with so great deliberation, giving them time and place whereby they might be changed from their wickedness:

With what circumspection hast thou judged thy own children, to whose parents thou hast sworn and made covenants of good promises?

Therefore whereas thou chastisest us, thou scourgest our enemies very many ways, to the end that when we judge we may think on thy goodness and when we are judged, we may hope for thy mercy.

Wherefore thou hast also greatly tormented them who in their life have lived foolishly and unjustly, by the same things which they worshipped.

For they went astray for a long time in the ways of error, holding those things for gods which are the most worthless among beasts, living after the manner of children without understanding.

Therefore thou hast sent a judgment upon them as senseless children to mock them.

But they that were not amended by mockeries and reprehensions, experienced the worthy judgment of God. For seeing with indignation that they suffered by those very things which they took for gods, when they were destroyed by the same, they acknowledged him the true God, whom in time past they denied that they knew for which cause the end also of their condemnation came upon them.

Chapter 13

But all men are vain, in whom there is not the knowledge of God and who by these good things that are seen, could not understand him that is, neither by attending to the works have

acknowledged who was the
workman

But have imagined either the fire,
or the wind, or the swift air, or
the circle of the stars, or the great
water, or the sun and moon, to be
the gods that rule the world.

With whose beauty, if they, being
delighted, took them to be gods
let them know how much the
Lord of them is more beautiful
than they for the first author of
beauty made all those things.

Or if they admired their power
and their effects, let them
understand by them, that he that

made them, is mightier than they.

For by the greatness of the beauty, and of the creature, the creator of them may be seen, so as to be known thereby.

But yet as to these they are less to be blamed.

For they perhaps err, seeking God, and desirous to find him.

For being conversant among his works, they search and they are persuaded that the things are good which are seen.

But then again they are not to be pardoned. For if they were able to know so much as to make a judgment of the world, how did they not more easily find out the Lord thereof?

But unhappy are they, and their hope is among the dead, who have called gods the works of the hands of men, gold and silver, the inventions of art, and the resemblances of beasts, or an unprofitable stone the work of an ancient hand.

Or if an artist, a carpenter, hath cut down a tree proper for his use in the wood and skillfully taken off all the bark thereof, and with his art, diligently formeth a vessel profitable for the common uses of life. And useth the chips of his work to dress his meat.

And taking what was left thereof, which is good for nothing, being a crooked piece of wood, and full of knots, carveth it diligently when he hath nothing else to do, and by the skill of his art fashioneth it and maketh it like the image of a man.

Or the resemblance of some beast, laying it over with vermilion, and painting it red, and covering every spot that is in it.

And maketh a convenient dwelling place for it, and setting it in a wall, and fastening it with iron, providing for it, lest it should fall, knowing that it is unable to help itself for it is an image, and hath need of help.

And then maketh prayer to it, inquiring concerning his substance, and his children, or his marriage. And he is not ashamed to speak to that which hath no life.

And for health he maketh supplication to the weak, and for life prayeth to that which is dead, and for help calleth upon that which is unprofitable.

And for a good journey he petitioneth him that cannot walk and for getting, and for working, and for the event of all things he asketh him that is unable to do any thing.

Chapter 14

Again, another designing to sail, and beginning to make his voyage through the raging waves, calleth upon a piece of wood more frail than the wood that carrieth him.

For this the desire of gain devised, and the workman built it by his skill.

But thy providence, O Father, governeth it for thou hast made a way even in the sea, and a most sure path among the waves, shewing that thou art able to save out of all things, yea though a man went to sea without art.

But that the works of thy wisdom might not be idle therefore, men also trust their lives even to a little wood, and passing over the sea by ship are saved.

And from the beginning also when the proud giants perished, the hope of the world fleeing to a vessel, which was governed by thy hand, left to the world seed of generation. For holy is the wood, by which justice cometh.

But the idol that is made by hands, is cursed, as well it, as he that made it.

He because he made it and it because being frail it is called a god.

But to God the wicked and his wickedness are hateful alike.

For that which is made, together with him that made it, shall suffer torments.

Therefore there shall be no respect had even to the idols of the Gentiles because the creatures of God are turned to an abomination, and a temptation to the souls of men, and a snare to the feet of the unwise.

For the beginning of fornication is the devising of idols and the invention of them is the corruption of life.

For neither were they from the beginning, neither shall they be forever.

For by the vanity of men they came into the world: and therefore they shall be found to come shortly to an end.

For a father being afflicted with bitter grief, made to himself the image of his son who was quickly taken away and him who then had died as a man, he began now to worship as a god and appointed him rites and sacrifices among his servants.

Then in process of time, wicked custom prevailing, this error was kept as a law, and statues were worshipped by the commandment of tyrants.

And those whom men could not honour in presence, because they dwelt far off, they brought their resemblance from afar, and made an express image of the king whom they had a mind to honour that by this their diligence, they might honour as present, him that was absent.

And to worshipping of these, the singular diligence also of the artificer helped to set forward the ignorant.

For he being willing to please him that employed him, laboured with all his art to make the resemblance in the best manner.

And the multitude of men, carried away by the beauty of the work, took him now for a god that a little before was but honoured as a man.

And this was the occasion of deceiving human life: for men serving either their affection, or their kings, gave the incommunicable name to stones and wood.

And it was not enough for them to err about the knowledge of God, but whereas they lived in a great war of ignorance, they call so many and so great evils peace.

For either they sacrifice their own children, or use hidden sacrifices, or keep watches full of madness. So that now they neither keep life, nor marriage undefiled, but one killeth another through envy, or grieveth him by adultery.

And all things are mingled together, blood, murder, theft and dissimulation, corruption and unfaithfulness, tumults and perjury, disquieting of the good,

Forgetfulness of God, defiling of souls, changing of nature, disorder in marriage, and the irregularity of adultery and uncleanness.

For the worship of abominable idols is the cause, and the beginning and end of all evil.

For either they are mad when they are merry or they prophesy lies, or they live unjustly or easily forswear themselves.

For whilst they trust in idols, which are without life, though they swear amiss, they look not to be hurt. But for two things they shall be justly punished, because they have thought not well of God, giving heed to idols, and have sworn unjustly, in guile despising justice.

For it is not the power of them, by whom they swear, but the just vengeance of sinners always punisheth the transgression of the unjust.

Chapter 15

But thou, our God, art gracious and true, patient, and ordering all things in mercy.

For if we sin, we are thine, knowing thy greatness and if we sin not, we know that we are counted with thee.

For to know thee is perfect justice: and to know thy justice, and thy power, is the root of immortality.

For the invention of mischievous men hath not deceived us, nor the shadow of a picture, a fruitless labour, a graven figure with divers colours.

The sight whereof enticeth the fool to lust after it, and he loveth the lifeless figure of a dead image.

The lovers of evil things deserve to have no better things to trust in, both they that make them, and they that love them, and they that worship them.

The potter also tempering soft earth, with labour fashioneth every vessel for our service, and of the same clay he maketh both vessels that are for clean uses, and likewise such as serve to the contrary but what is the use of these vessels, the potter is the judge.

And of the same clay by a vain labour he maketh a god, he who a little before was made of earth himself, and a little after returneth to the same out of which he was taken, when his life which was lent him shall be called for again.

But his care is, not that he shall labour, nor that his life is short, but he striveth with the goldsmiths and silversmiths, and he endeavoureth to do like the workers in brass, and counteth it a glory to make vain things.

For his heart is ashes, and his hope vain earth, and his life more base than clay:

Forasmuch as he knew not his maker and him that inspired into him the soul that worketh, and that breathed into him a living spirit.

Yea and they have counted our life a pastime, and the business of life to be gain, and that we must be getting every way, even out of evil.

For that man knoweth that he offendeth above all others, who of earthly matter maketh brittle vessels, and graven gods.

But all the enemies of thy people that hold them in subjection, are foolish, and unhappy, and proud beyond measure.

For they have esteemed all the idols of the heathens for gods, which neither have the use of eyes to see, nor noses to draw breath, nor ears to hear, nor fingers of hands to handle, and as for their feet, they are slow to walk.

For man made them and he that borroweth his own breath, fashioned them.

For no man can make a god like to himself.

For being mortal himself, he formeth a dead thing with his wicked hands. For he is better than they whom he worshippeth, because he indeed hath lived, though he were mortal, but they never.

Moreover they worship also the vilest creatures: but things

without sense compared to these, are worse than they.

Yea, neither by sight can any man see good of these beasts. But they have fled from the praise of God, and from his blessing.

Chapter 16

For these things, and by the like things to these, they were worthily punished, and were destroyed by a multitude of beasts.

Instead of which punishment, dealing well with thy people, thou gavest them their desire of delicious food, of a new taste, preparing for them quails for their meat.

To the end that they indeed desiring food, by means of those things that were shewn and sent among them, might loathe even that which was necessary to satisfy their desire.

But these, after suffering want for a short time, tasted a new meat. For it was requisite that inevitable destruction should come upon them that exercised tyranny but to these it should only be shewn how their enemies were destroyed.

For when the fierce rage of beasts came upon these, they were destroyed with the bitings of crooked serpents.

But thy wrath endured not forever, but they were troubled for a short time for their correction, having a sign of salvation to put them in remembrance of the commandment of thy law.

For he that turned to it, was not healed by that which he saw, but by thee the Saviour of all.

And in this thou didst shew to our enemies, that thou art he who deliverest from all evil.

For the bitings of locusts, and of flies killed them, and there was found no remedy for their life: because they were worthy to be destroyed by such things.

But not even the teeth of venomous serpents overcame thy children for thy mercy came and healed them.

For they were examined for the remembrance of thy words, and were quickly healed, lest falling into deep forgetfulness, they might not be able to use thy help.

For it was neither herb, nor mollifying plaster that healed

them, but thy word, O Lord, which healeth all things.

For it is thou, O Lord, that hast power of life and death, and leadest down to the gates of death, and bringest back again.

A man indeed killeth through malice, and when the spirit is gone forth, it shall not return, neither shall he call back the soul that is received.

But it is impossible to escape thy hand. For the wicked that denied to know thee, were scourged by the strength of thy arm, being persecuted by strange waters, and hail, and rain, and consumed by fire.

And which was wonderful, in water, which extinguisheth all things, the fire had more force: for the world fighteth for the just.

For at one time, the fire was mitigated, that the beasts which were sent against the wicked might not be burned, but that they might see and perceive that they were persecuted by the judgment of God.

And at another time the fire, above its own power, burned in the midst of water, to destroy the fruits of a wicked land.

Instead of which things thou didst feed thy people with the food of angels, and gavest them bread from heaven prepared without labour having in it all that is delicious, and the sweetness of every taste.

For thy sustenance shewed thy sweetness to thy children, and serving every man's will, it was turned to what every man liked.

But snow and ice endured the force of fire, and melted not: that they might know that fire burning in the hail and flashing in the rain destroyed the fruits of the enemies.

But this same again, that the just might be nourished, did even forget its own strength.

For the creature serving thee the Creator, is made fierce against the unjust for their punishment and abateth its strength for the benefit of them that trust in thee.

Therefore even then it was transformed into all things, and was obedient to thy grace that nourisheth all, according to the will of them that desired it of thee.

That thy children, O Lord, whom thou lovedst, might know that it is not the growing of fruits that nourisheth men, but thy word preserveth them that believe in thee.

For that which could not be destroyed by fire, being warmed with a little sunbeam presently melted away.

That it might be known to all, that we ought to prevent the sun to bless thee, and adore thee at the dawning of the light.

For the hope of the unthankful shall melt away as the winter's ice, and shall run off as unprofitable water.

Chapter 17

For thy judgments, O Lord, are great, and thy words cannot be expressed therefore undisciplined souls have erred.

For while the wicked thought to be able to have dominion over the holy nation, they themselves being fettered with the bonds of darkness, and a long night, shut up in their houses, lay there exiled from the eternal providence.

And while they thought to lie hid in their obscure sins, they were scattered under a dark veil of forgetfulness, being horribly afraid and troubled with exceeding great astonishment.

For neither did the den that held them, keep them from fear: for noises coming down troubled them, and sad visions appearing to them, affrighted them.

And no power of fire could give them light, neither could the bright flames of the stars enlighten that horrible night.

But there appeared to them a sudden fire, very dreadful: and being struck with the fear of that face, which was not seen, they thought the things which they saw to be worse.

And the delusions of their magic art were put down, and their boasting of wisdom was reproachfully rebuked.

For they who promised to drive away fears and troubles from a sick soul, were sick themselves of a fear worthy to be laughed at.

For though no terrible thing disturbed them: yet being scared with the passing by of beasts, and hissing of serpents, they died for fear: and denying that they saw the air, which could by no means be avoided.

For whereas wickedness is fearful, it beareth witness of its condemnation for a troubled conscience always forecasteth grievous things.

For fear is nothing else but a yielding up of the succours from thought.

And while there is less expectation from within, the greater doth it count the ignorance of that cause which bringeth the torment.

But they that during that night, in which nothing could be done, and which came upon them from the lowest and deepest hell, slept the same sleep.

Were sometimes molested with the fear of monsters, sometimes fainted away, their soul failing them: for a sudden and unlooked for fear was come upon them.

Moreover if any of them had fallen down, he was kept shut up in prison without irons.

For if any one were a husbandman, or a shepherd, or a labourer in the field, and was suddenly overtaken, he endured a necessity from which he could not fly.

For they were all bound together with one chain of darkness.

Whether it were a whistling wind, or the melodious voice of birds, among the spreading branches of trees, or a fall of water running down with violence.

Or the mighty noise of stones tumbling down, or the running that could not be seen of beasts playing together, or the roaring voice of wild beasts, or a rebounding echo from the highest mountains these things made them to swoon for fear.

For the whole world was enlightened with a clear light, and none were hindered in their labours.

But over them only was spread a heavy night, an image of that darkness which was to come upon them. But they were to themselves more grievous than the darkness.

Chapter 18

But thy saints had a very great light, and they heard their voice indeed, but did not see their shape. And because they also did not suffer the same things, they glorified thee.

And they that before had been wronged, gave thanks, because they were not hurt now and asked this gift, that there might be a difference.

Therefore they received a burning pillar of fire for a guide of the way which they knew not, and thou gavest them a harmless sun of a good entertainment.

The others indeed were worthy to be deprived of light, and imprisoned in darkness, who kept thy children shut up, by whom the pure light of the law was to be given to the world.

And whereas they thought to kill the babes of the just, one child being cast forth, and saved, to reprove them, thou tookest away a multitude of their children, and destroyedst them all together in a mighty water.

For that night was known before by our fathers, that assuredly knowing what oaths they had trusted to, they might be of better courage.

So thy people received the salvation of the just, and destruction of the unjust.

For as thou didst punish the adversaries: so thou didst also encourage and glorify us.

For the just children of good men were offering sacrifice secretly, and they unanimously ordered a law of justice that the just should receive both good and evil alike, singing now the praises of the fathers.

But on the other side there sounded an ill according cry of the enemies, and a lamentable mourning was heard for the children that were bewailed.

And the servant suffered the same punishment as the master, and a common man suffered in like manner as the king.

So all alike had innumerable dead, with one kind of death.

Neither were the living sufficient to bury them; for in one moment the noblest offspring of them was destroyed.

For whereas they would not believe any thing before by reason of the enchantments, then first upon the destruction of the firstborn, they acknowledged the people to be of God.

For while all things were in quiet silence, and the night was in the midst of her course thy almighty word leapt down from heaven from thy royal throne, as a fierce conqueror into the midst of the land of destruction.

With a sharp sword carrying thy unfeigned commandment, and he stood and filled all things with death, and standing on the earth reached even to heaven.

Then suddenly visions of evil dreams troubled them, and fears unlooked for came upon them.

And one thrown here, another there, half dead, shewed the cause of his death.

For the visions that troubled them foreshewed these things, lest they should perish and not know why they suffered these evils.

But the just also were afterwards touched by an assault of death, and there was a disturbance of the multitude in the wilderness but thy wrath did not long continue.

For a blameless man made haste to pray for the people, bringing forth the shield of his ministry, prayer, and by incense making supplication, withstood the wrath, and put an end to the calamity, shewing that he was thy servant.

And he overcame the disturbance, not by strength of body nor with force of arms, but with a word he subdued him that punished them, alleging the oaths and covenant made with the fathers.

For when they were now fallen down dead by heaps one upon another, he stood between and stayed the assault, and cut off the way to the living.

For in the priestly robe which he wore, was the whole world and in the four rows of the stones the glory of the fathers was graven, and thy majesty was written upon the diadem of his head. And to these the destroyer gave place, and was afraid of them: for the proof only of wrath was enough.

Chapter 19

But as to the wicked, even to the end there came upon them wrath without mercy. For he knew before also what they would do.

For when they had given them leave to depart, and had sent them away with great care, they repented, and pursued after them.

For whilst they were yet mourning, and lamenting at the graves of the dead, they took up another foolish device and pursued them as fugitives whom they had pressed to be gone.

For a necessity, of which they were worthy, brought them to this end and they lost the remembrance of those things which had happened, that their punishment might fill up what was wanting to their torments.

And that thy people might wonderfully pass through, but they might find a new death.

For every creature according to its kind was fashioned again as from the beginning, obeying thy commandments, that thy children might be kept without hurt.

For a cloud overshadowed their camp, and where water was before, dry land appeared, and in the Red Sea a way without hinderance, and out of the great deep a springing field.

Through which all the nation passed which was protected with thy hand, seeing thy miracles and wonders.

For they fed on their food like horses, and they skipped like lambs, praising thee, O Lord, who hadst delivered them.

For they were yet mindful of those things which had been done in the time of their sojourning, how the ground brought forth flies instead of cattle, and how the river cast up a multitude of frogs instead of fishes.

And at length they saw a new generation of birds, when being led by their appetite they asked for delicate meats.

For to satisfy their desire, the quail came up to them from the sea: and punishments came upon the sinners, not without foregoing signs by the force of thunders: for they suffered justly according to their own wickedness.

For they exercised a more detestable inhospitality than any others indeed received not strangers unknown to them, but these brought their guests into bondage that had deserved well of them.

And not only so, but in another respect also they were worse for the others against their will received the strangers.

But these grievously afflicted them whom they had received with joy, and who lived under the same laws.

But they were struck with blindness as those others were at the doors of the just man, when they were covered with sudden darkness, and every one sought the passage of his own door.

For while the elements are changed in themselves, as in an instrument the sound of the quality is changed, yet all keep their sound: which may clearly be perceived by the very sight.

For the things of the land were turned into things of the water: and the things before swam in the water passed upon the land.

The fire had power in water above its own virtue, and the water forgot its quenching nature.

On the other side, the flames wasted not the flesh of corruptible animals walking therein, neither did they melt that good food, which was apt to melt as ice. For in all things thou didst magnify thy people, O Lord, and didst honour them, and didst not despise them, but didst assist them at all times, and in every place.

CLOSING WORDS

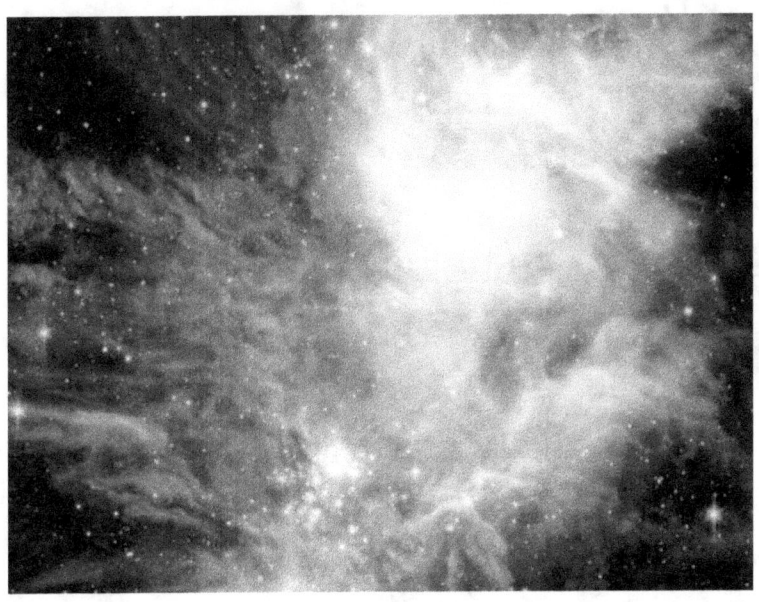

By having completed this work, you have began the most important step of your life and wisdom will be yours by learning to win against the battle of iniquity upon your life.

In conclusion here is an excerpt taught by Christ Yeshu, from the Ancient Word Series: The Gospel of Peace:

THE ANGEL OF WISDOM

To follow the Lord
Is the beginning of Wisdom:
And the knowledge
Of the Holy One
Is understanding.
For by him
Thy days shall be multiplied,
And the years of thy life
Shall be increased.
All Wisdom cometh from the
Heavenly Father, Yehowah,

And is with him forever.
Through the holy Law doth the
Angel of Wisdom
Guide the Children of Light.
Who can number the sand of the
sea, And the drops Of rain, and
the days of eternity? Who can
find out the height of heaven,
And the breadth of the earth,
And the deep, and wisdom?
Wisdom hath been
created before all things.
One may heal with goodness,
One may heal with justice,
One may heal with herbs,
One may heal
with the Wise Word.
Amongst all the remedies,
This one is the healing one
That heals with the Wise Word.
And one it is that will

best drive away sickness
From the bodies of the faithful,
For Wisdom is the best healing of
all remedies. To follow the holy
Law is the crown of Wisdom,
Making peace and
perfect health to flourish,
Both which are the gifts of the
Angels. We would
draw near unto thee,
O Heavenly Father, Yehowah!
With the help of thy Angel of
Wisdom, Who guides us by
means of thy Heavenly Order,
And with the actions and the
words inspired
by thy holy Wisdom!
Come to us, Heavenly Father,
Yehowah, with
thy creative mind.

And do thou, who bestoweth gifts
through thy Heavenly Order,
Bestow alike the
longlasting gift of Wisdom
Upon the Children of Light, that
this life might be
spent in holy service in the
Garden of the Brotherhood.
In the realm of thy good mind,
Incarnate in our minds, The path
of Wisdom doth flow from the
Heavenly Order,
Wherein doth dwell the sacred
Tree of Life. In what fashion is
manifest thy Law,
O Heavenly Father, Yehowah!
The Heavenly Father, Yehowah
makes answer:
By good thought
In perfect unity with
Wisdom, O Child of Light!

What is the word well spoken?
It is the benevolent
bestowing word of Wisdom.
What is the thought well thought?
It is that which the
Child of Light thinketh,
The one who holdeth
the Holy Thought
To be the most of value
of all things else.
So shall the Child of Light grow
In concentration and
communion, And he may
develop Wisdom,
And thus shall he continue
Until all the mysteries of the
Infinite Garden
Where standeth the Tree of Life
Shall be revealed to him.
Then shall he say
these victorious words:

O Heavenly Father, Yehowah!
Give unto me my task
For the building
of thy Kingdom on earth,
Through good thoughts, good
words, good deeds,
Which shall be for
thy child of Light
His and her most precious gift.
O thou Heavenly Order!
And thou Universal Mind!
I will worship thee and the
Heavenly Father, Yehowah,
Because of whom
the creative mind within us
Is causing the Imperishable
Kingdom to progress!
Holy Wisdom maketh all men
free from fear,
Wide of heart, and easy of
conscience.

Holy Wisdom, the
understanding
that unfolds forever,
Continually, without end,
And is not acquired
through the holy scrolls.
It is ignorance that
ruineth most people,
Both amongst those
who have died, And those who
shall die. When ignorance will be
replaced by Holy Wisdom,
Then will sweetness and
fatness come back again
To our land and to our fields,
With health and healing,
With fullness and
increase, and growth,
And abundance of
corn and of grass,

And rivers of Peace shall flow
through the desert.

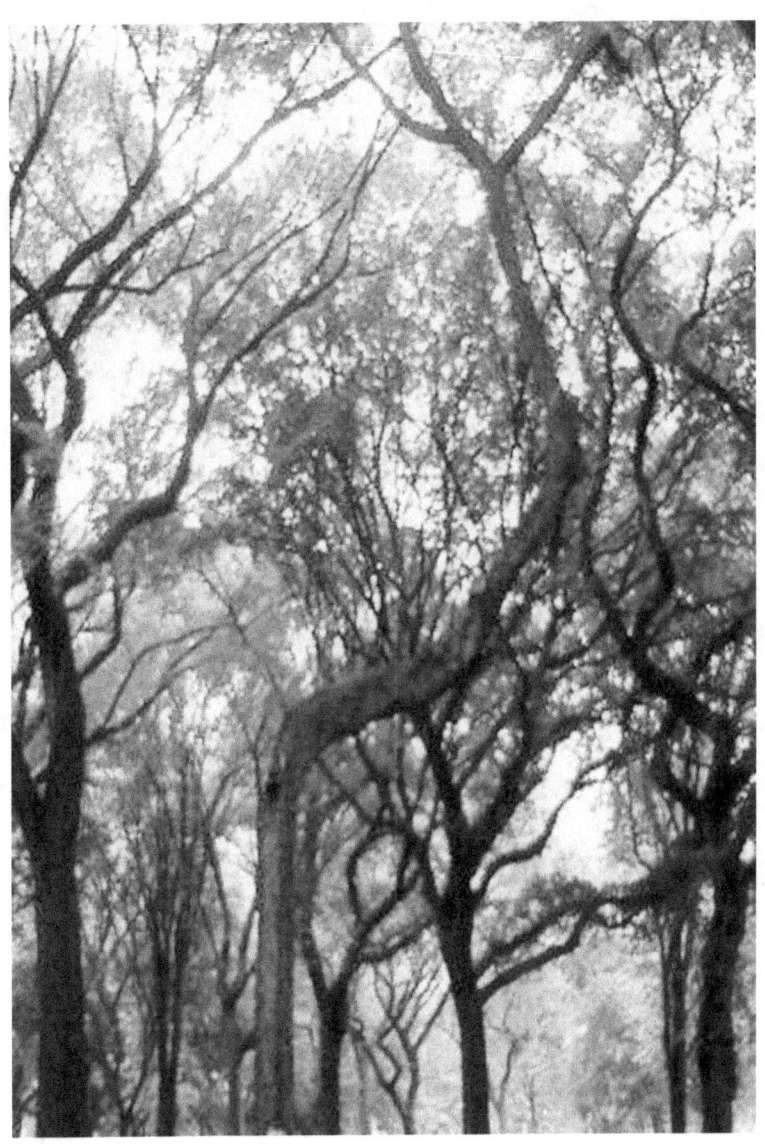

In Wisdom, Peace and Love,
Peace be always with thee.

Rev. Melissa Smith

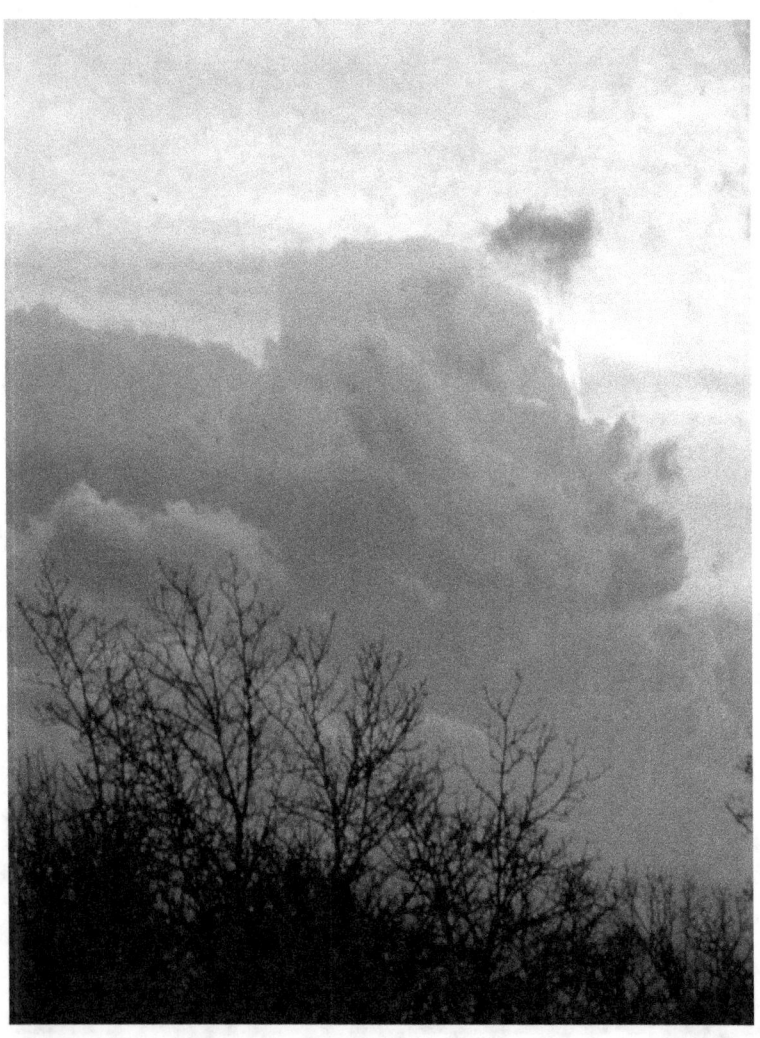